TOP 5 FOODS FOR MEN TO INCREASE FERTILITY

How to Boost Sperm

MICHELLE C. ROBINSON

All rights reserved. No part of this publication may be reproduced, distributed, or transmitted in any form or by any means, including photocopying, recording, or other electronic or mechanical methods, without the prior written permission of the publisher, except in the case of brief quotations embodied in critical reviews and certain other noncommercial uses permitted by copyright law.

Copyright © (Michelle C. Robinson), (2022).

Contents

Chapter 1: Various Techniques For Analyzing Men's Fertility, Male Infertility Test, Analysis of Sperm And Semen, Antibodies Against Sperm, Viagra Could Affect Men's Fertility

Chapter 2: Five Supplements to Improve Male Fertility

Chapter 3: Male Infertility Cure And Treatment, Causes of Male Infertility, Consume Meals That Can Aid in Increasing Sperm Cell Production, Herbs And Oils That Can Boost Sperm Production

Chapter 4: Top Five Foods For Men to Increase Fertility, Ten Strategies to Boost Male Fertility

Chapter 5: Conclusion

Introduction

So, you're prepared to become a parent. After consulting your doctor, you have stopped taking medicines and begun taking those folic acid supplements. Unfortunately, you are still unable to get pregnant. If so, it might be time to figure out how to make your mate more fertile. After all, it takes two to conceive.

Before doing anything else, you and your partner should visit a doctor to find out whether there are any hidden medical reasons for your or your partner's infertility. It is undoubtedly essential to get medical conditions treated as soon as possible if they are present. If not, you should probably look into natural approaches to boosting fertility.

Low sperm count is typically to blame in men. Fortunately, increasing sperm production is simple, though it can take some time to see benefits. For starters, males whose testicles are exposed to extreme temperatures typically have low sperm counts. You should advise your partner to wear cotton boxers rather than briefs to resolve this issue. He should also start abstaining from hot baths and saunas, as these activities may further reduce sperm production. About this, you two should use the fact that sperm counts are higher in the morning, which is likely one of the best times to try for a child.

By controlling the frequency of your sex sessions, you and your spouse can learn how to boost fertility. If your partner's sperm count is poor, he should only ejaculate two or three times each week. Instead, he should be ejaculating more frequently—roughly every one to two days—if his issue is due to the poor quality of his sperm.

Encourage him to lead a better lifestyle as another approach to boost your partner's fertility. He should give up any vices, such as smoking and using drugs, as quickly as feasible. Along with quitting drinking alcohol, he should start consuming less caffeine. A healthy diet and regular exercise might also work wonders for his fertility.

As long as your spouse and you are devoted to learning how to boost fertility, getting pregnant is not difficult.

Chapter 1

Various Techniques for Analyzing Men's Fertility

Even though nearly half of all cases of infertility involve issues with men, many people still view it as a "female problem." The decreased fertility of men is to blame for about 20–30% of cases of infertility. Given this information, males must get tested for reduced fertility, along with their partners. Some people may find this quite embarrassing, yet early testing equals early treatment and a successful pregnancy. By getting checked, you can prevent your partner from experiencing unneeded suffering.

Preliminary analysis of male infertility

If you haven't conceived a kid following a year of frequent, uncovered sex, many doctors will find a diagnosis of infertility. However, a more accurate diagnosis would be impaired infertility because most couples can conceive if they attempt for at least a year after the first. An evaluation for male infertility should start with a visit to a urologist if you can still conceive after three years.

A physical examination and an interview are the first steps in this procedure. A thorough reproductive and medical history is required, as well as a record of the medications you have been taking and any policies you may have.

Additionally, questions about your lifestyle, such as whether or not you smoke, exercise, or use drugs, will be asked of you. You must be open and honest about your sexual life, including any STDs or other issues. Additionally, your urologist will need a sample of your semen for infertility testing.

Male infertility tests

Once your infertility has been identified, the next step is determining what caused it. Although approaches taken by specialists typically vary, you can anticipate the following tests: To measure the size of your testicles and identify any varicoceles or hormonal issues, a thorough physical examination, ideally by a urologist, is necessary. Sperm and semen analysis is also recommended. Because testosterone and other hormones regulate sperm production in your body, your doctor may also advise you to get a hormonal evaluation. But according to experts, hormonal imbalances do not account for most cases of male infertility. Genetic testing can identify the causes of male infertility, such as sperm quality issues.

Analysis of sperm and semen

Your urologist will evaluate your sperm count along with other factors like the movement and shape of your sperm during a thorough sperm and semen analysis. You are probably more fertile if most of your sperm have a standard form. Many men are fertile despite having abnormal sperm or a low sperm count. Approximately 15% of male infertility cases are unrelated to low sperm counts or unusually shaped semen. Your doctor might request that you undergo testing again if the results of your sperm and semen analysis are expected to be sure. Two average test results, however, do not guarantee that you do not experience infertility. If your doctor notices a discrepancy in the test results, you might be asked to undergo additional testing to pinpoint the issue. If you have azoospermia (the absence of sperm or semen), it may be caused by a blockage that can resolve surgically.

Antibodies against sperm

Some men's abnormal antibodies attack the sperm as it travels to the egg, preventing fertilization. In these circumstances, the sperm count is typically average, but the semen is mainly devoid of sperm. There are several potential causes for average sperm counts that do not manifest in semen, including retrograde ejaculation, the absence of the sperm pipeline, obstructions between the penis and the testicles, and others.

The majority of couples who experience infertility issues determine the cause through testing. In most cases of male infertility, a proper diagnosis and course of treatment are effective.

Viagra Could Affect Men's Fertility

Men who take Viagra run the risk of having lower fertility. Many prospective fathers who have been regularly consuming Viagra for improved sexual performance would undoubtedly receive a nasty shock from the findings of the most recent study on the drug's impact on sperm motility and lifespan. Before using erectile dysfunction medication, men may require some time to assess the benefits and drawbacks of the side effects of taking Viagra.

The anti-impotence medicine Viagra speeds up sperm and causes the crucial response required to pierce an egg to occur early, according to David Glenn, one of the pioneers on the Queen's University team that carried out the test tube studies in Belfast, Northern Ireland. It is true that the majority of men who use Viagra do so because they are impotent, and most of them are middle-aged men who have no plans to have children. It might not be a problem for users in this category.

If they have plans to become fathers in the near or distant future, the growing number of young men and women who use Viagra for erectile dysfunction may want to reconsider their use of the drug. Additionally, a lot of teenagers who use Viagra recreationally may later come to regret their bad choices.

The research team collected 45 samples of semen from men visiting a reproductive clinic, gave half of them Viagra, and kept the other half for a carefully controlled trial When a man consumed a 100ml. Pill of

Viagra, the dose concentration was clinically determined to be equivalent to the level of Viagra in blood plasma if you discovered that the sperm treated with Viagra began to accelerate in 15 seconds flat and continued for around 135 seconds.

After two hours of observation, you will also discover that in the Viagra samples, compared to the controlled trial, around 79% more sperm were in a wholly responded state. Digestive enzymes are released from the sperm's head during this acrosome process, which is necessary for a sperm to enter an egg and fertilize it. The method of fertilization may suffer from the sperm's early reaction.

Phosphodiesterase, an enzyme that aids in the breakdown of messenger molecules related to energy production, is inhibited by sildenafil, the primary active ingredient of Viagra. Inhibiting energy breakdown causes the energy level in cells to rise, resulting in increased sperm motility, which can be detrimental to the embryo's growth. If someone wants to leave behind descendants, using Viagra is most certainly not necessary.

It is past time for Viagra users to understand the terrible repercussions of using the drug for amusement and frivolity. Take Viagra with a grain of salt to produce descendants worth their salt.

Chapter 2

Five Supplements to Improve Male Fertility

A lot of couples hope to have kids in the future. Unfortunately, despite their best efforts, many of them fail to reproduce. Sometimes a man may need assistance because of a problem with his fertility. Men who want to increase their fertility chances should focus on maintaining a healthy diet and lifestyle. Vitamins and specific foods are excellent sources for enhancing male fertility. The top five vitamins that help boost male fertility are listed below.

Vitamin C

The most significant ways to boost sperm count are with vitamins for infertility, and Vitamin C is a fantastic place to start. Many fruits and foods, including mango, oranges, kiwi, broccoli, peppers, and potatoes, contain vitamin C. This vitamin increases sperm flow and prevents clumping, increasing a man's fertility probability. Because studies have indicated that vitamin C helps promote male fertility, so men should consume 500–1,000 mg daily.

Vitamin E

Because vitamin E gives sperm the strength to enter the woman's egg, it will boost male fertility. The most crucial step in conception is this. The best sources of vitamin E include cereal, sunflower seeds, nuts, green leafy vegetables, tomatoes, peanut butter, and avocados. The suggested daily dose is 15 mg, although the body won't suffer if you take more. Vitamin E supplementation will boost male fertility.

Vitamin B

One of many vitamins that can increase male fertility is vitamin B, particularly vitamin B12. B12 has no upper intake limit since, even at high levels, it has no adverse effects on the body. However, 2.4 mcg is the suggested daily dose. It can be used as a supplement and improves sperm production and quality. Fish, beans, eggs, seafood, milk, and leafy green vegetables are good sources of vitamin B12 and other B vitamins.

Arginine

The effectiveness of vitamins for infertility has been demonstrated, and arginine is no exception. This amino acid boosts sperm quality and quantity. The couple's chances of getting pregnant increase with the amount of sperm ejaculated. It is advised to consume four milligrams every day. Foods high in arginine include cheese, milk, yogurt, chicken, pork, seafood, oats, and almonds.

Zinc

Men need a lot of zinc because they lose five milligrams of it with each ejaculation. He must boost his regular zinc consumption to compensate for his loss. Additionally, zinc is known to increase sperm count and motility and protect DNA from harm. Because studies reveal that infertile men lack zinc,

zinc is one of the essential vitamins for infertility. Good sources of zinc include oysters, yogurt, cashews, pine nuts, milk, cheese, and oats. For health, one to four milligrams of zinc per day are sufficient.

Everyday meals that support a healthy and reproductive body are known as fertility foods. Among the best foods for boosting male fertility are dairy products, salmon, meat, yams, berries, and oysters. The best thing men can do to increase their fertility is to eat a well-balanced diet rich in vitamins and minerals. Several fertility foods promise to help make men fertile. They can consider vitamin supplements if they cannot obtain these vitamins from their regular meals to increase fertility.

However, speak with your doctor or physician to go through your alternatives and strategies to increase your fertility before changing your diet or taking any vitamins.

Chapter 3

Male Infertility Cure And Treatment - Some Tips on How to Improve Fertility in Men

The topic of increasing male fertility is often discussed and well-known. According to statistics, between 30 and 40 percent of couples experience difficulties throughout pregnancy and childbearing. Males who underwent fertility testing had low sperm counts or aberrant, immature sperm in the results. Premature ejaculation and impotence can occasionally make it difficult to get pregnant. It is best to get a fertility study for both partners when the couple has made multiple tries, but pregnancy has not occurred. Following consultation and a comprehensive review of the circumstances, will perform the test as per the doctor's prescription.

Causes of Male Infertility

Men can become infertile for many reasons, including some of the following as follows:

The disorder known as varicocele causes dilated scrotal veins. Blood flow is obstructed as a result, which results in the development of immature sperm cells. Can use Medical techniques to treat varicocele.

Low sperm production, sperm production that is immature or aberrant, or even no sperm production can all contribute to infertility.

Because sperm are discharged earlier and are produced more quickly, premature ejaculation might result in infertility because the sperm are of lower quality. The weakening of the muscles brought on by disorders of the neurological system or other conditions results in premature ejaculation.

There is an obstruction in the sperm's pathway.

Hormonal dysregulation

Issues with the genetic makeup

Negative effects of cancer

Being exposed to heat

Drug and alcohol abuse are both problems.

1. Smoking

People living with Male infertility don't have to be depressed because they can effectively manage these illnesses. It can also avoid The predisposing variables to reach a good state of well-being. For couples who want to become pregnant, there are many options accessible. In-vitro fertilization, IVF, and intracytoplasmic sperm injection are examples of such procedures. A healthy newborn can be delivered to prospective parents using these two tried-and-true techniques. Books are a fantastic way to learn about enhancing male fertility.

The following suggestions will help you produce more sperm cells.

2. Maintaining a fit lifestyle

Factual fertility enhancement begins with a healthy lifestyle. It would be ideal to consume nutrient-dense foods that are sufficiently mineral- and vitamin-rich. Regular exercise is another thing you should think about doing to keep your body physically fit. Maintaining mental and physical focus will also support good health.

3. Consume meals that can aid in increasing sperm cell production.

Antioxidant-rich foods, such as fruits and vegetables, are unquestionably wise because they boost sperm cell development. Apples are a great source of antioxidants and can help men produce more sperm. You would benefit if you were conscious of your nutrition because it significantly impacts your fertility. Vitamins and other dietary supplements can also greatly aid in increasing fertility. Vitamins C and E are two things you should consider taking. You should also consider including zinc and selenium in your diet.

Herbs and oils that can boost sperm production

Many oils and herbs that are readily sold on the market can be used to aid in boosting sperm count. These herbs include palmetto, astral Gus, macaw, and Chinese ginseng, to name a few. In addition to these herbs, various oils, such as flax seed oil, pumpkin seed oil, sunflower oil, and some fish oils, can aid in boosting the number of sperm. Additionally, there are several over-the-counter drugs like Viagra that assist with male infertility issues. Males should visit their doctor before taking these oils, herbs, or other drugs to prevent significant adverse effects.

Remember that preparation is necessary for a healthy pregnancy and newborn. Living a healthy lifestyle throughout this stage of pregnancy, such as engaging in regular exercise, would be an excellent place to start. Remember to take frequent breaks from work to unwind and relieve tension.

Chapter 4

Top 5 Foods for Men to Increase Fertility

First, men are responsible for roughly 40% of all fertility issues. Age or poor health might affect a man's fertility. A nutritionally balanced diet is essential for overall health as well as fertility.

According to research, poor dietary practices are directly related to poor sperm quality and low sperm counts. For instance, males who consume fewer fruits and vegetables are more prone to experience this issue.

But eating these things can increase your likelihood of getting pregnant:

Asparagus

It is a vegetable that may increase sperm production. In the past, used this frequently used vegetable to treat infertility. Additionally, it has a significant amount of vitamin C, which improves the viability and motility of sperm. This delicious veggie is best consumed as a salad.

Banana

Magnesium, vitamin A, B1, vitamin C, and protein are abundant in this well-liked option and necessary for increased sperm production. Bromelain, a potent regulator of sexual hormones that can help increase virility, is great in this fruit. Eat bananas as part of your everyday diet. While enjoying its advantages and boost, you can also cook banana shakes and smoothies.

Cacao Nuts

Short-term zinc deficiency can lower sperm volume and impact testosterone levels. Cashew nuts contain a lot of zinc. Men's fertility and good health both depend on zinc, a mineral. Additionally, it is thought to raise testosterone levels. If you include cashew nuts in your diet, a few handfuls won't harm you.

Garlic

It includes selenium and vitamin B6, making it a well-known superfood for sexual health. Selenium is a mineral that fights oxidation, increases sexual virility, and prevents sperm damage, while vitamin B6 strengthens the immune system and controls hormones. Allicin, abundant in garlic and helps to get great erections by increasing blood flow to the sexual organs, is an excellent source of allicin. For maximum results, add minced garlic to your favorite dishes.

Oysters

Additionally, oysters are a fantastic source of zinc, which contributes to the formation of the sperm's tail and outer layer. A daily dose of 15mg of oysters can assist in strengthening and improving sperm that have been harmed by toxins absorbed from the environment.

You can get plenty of zinc from nuts, beans, seeds, eggs, etc., if you can't afford or stomach oysters.

Ten Strategies to Boost Male Fertility

You are not alone if you and your partner have trouble getting pregnant. More than 6 million people each year experience difficulties getting pregnant, and this figure is steadily increasing. There are several cases of infertility. It impacts people of all ages, races, socioeconomic statuses, and sexes. However, there are steps you may take to improve your fertility if you are experiencing male infertility, which a low sperm count and irregular sperm production typically bring on. There are strategies to increase your chances of conception.

Here are Ten scientifically supported methods for sperm enhancement.

1. Eat More Folate-Rich Foods

Not only are pregnant women in need of folic acid, but so are their spouses. A University of California, Berkeley study claims that individuals with decreased dietary folic acid intake had a higher incidence of defective chromosomes in their sperm. The fertilization of an egg by sperm with faulty chromosomes may cause miscarriage or birth abnormalities. (Chromosome abnormalities in the embryo are to blame for more than half of miscarriages in the first trimester.)

How can you then include folic acid in your diet? Supplements are an option, but your best bet is to eat more folate foods, such as beans, whole grains, leafy greens, citrus fruits, cereals, bread, and kinds of pasta fortified with the vitamin.

2. Obtained Enough Sleep

Researchers at Aarhus University in Denmark connected earlier bedtimes with better sperm quality in a 2019 study. They were going to bed before 10:30 p.m. is the key. The researchers also identified a correlation between obtaining sufficient sleep—between seven-and-a-half and eight hours each night—with enhanced fertility.

3. Take a Male Fertility Supplement Right Away

Because it takes two to make an embryo, both partners should think about taking prenatal vitamins. "There is no disadvantage in staying as healthy as possible while attempting to conceive with your spouse," says Selenium. "Selenium has been demonstrated to lessen the incidence of birth abnormalities and improve low sperm counts."

4. Quit smoking to hasten sperm movement

Another justification for quitting smoking has been added to your comparative report's "why to quit" column: smoking can result in poor sperm counts and slow-moving sperm. At least three months should pass before you try to get pregnant. Changes you make today won't manifest in the semen for at least three months, according to Sperm production takes roughly three months. You should also avoid Marijuana and other illegal drugs because they may harm sperm. When couples use recreational drugs like cocaine, Marijuana, or other common amphetamines, the risk of miscarriage also rises.

5. Limit alcohol consumption to prevent abnormal sperm.

While you don't have to give it up totally, it's a good idea to limit your alcohol intake if you're trying to conceive. It has been demonstrated that alcohol decreases sperm production and produces defective sperm.

6. Set up a pre-conception examination

Before attempting conception, it is a good idea to have a complete physical examination to understand your health and fertility better. Expect to talk about your genetic history, weight, medication use, lifestyle choices, and what you can do to have a good pregnancy. Additionally, vaccinations may be given to you to help shield you from contracting diseases like Chickenpox and the seasonal flu while pregnant.

7. Reduce Caffeine to Increase Sperm Count

A study of Danish men discovered that men who consumed a lot of soda and caffeine had somewhat lower sperm counts and concentrations. Dr. John advises limiting your daily caffeine intake to 300 mg, or about three 6-ounce portions, which includes coffee, tea, chocolate, and energy drinks.

8. Lose Stress Through Exercise

Stress can decrease sperm concentration and increase aberrant sperm.
You can manage stress by getting enough rest, eating a healthy diet, exercising frequently, and doing other fun activities.

9. Verify That Your Medicines Are Fertility-Friendly

Before trying to conceive, note all the medications you are currently taking, such as vitamins, herbal supplements, prescription drugs, and over-the-counter drugs. You should also see your doctor.

Some medicines may have an impact on your sperm's number or quality. Your doctor should be able to suggest a more fertility-friendly alternative if you're taking a prescription that can potentially interfere with your plans to have children.

10. Consume more nuts

Research demonstrating the connection between walnuts and fertility was published in October 2013 in the Biology of Reproduction Papers-in-Press. Notably, it showed that consuming 75 grams of walnuts per day enhanced "sperm viability, motility, and morphology"—possibly due to the antioxidants, vitamins, and alpha-linolenic acid (ALA) walnuts contain.

Chapter 5

Conclusion

Advice on How to Approach Men About Infertility

About 7.3 million American women of reproductive age have sought reproductive services (1), occasionally with less than accommodating partners. The differing ways that men and women tackle infertility can strain relationships. It may be possible for women to reestablish harmony and the shared effort of attempting to conceive by considering why men are reluctant to undergo reproductive treatment.

So why would a man dispute the initial need for assistance? Women are frequently more accepting of medical testing of any kind and might not see anything wrong with getting looked out for, especially if the test is one that their insurance would pay for. Men may sometimes view it differently.

The challenge of scheduling an appointment and delivering the semen samples to the lab comes first. Men frequently don't want to go to the clinic and take a semen sample because it can be awkward. Men may find it very unsettling to use the collecting room, which is typically a restroom with some pornographic publications, especially if the walls are not soundproof and they can hear people nearby conversing or strolling by. Some males find it intimidating to "act on demand," which raises their stress levels. Asking the clinic if men can submit their specimens at home is helpful. A man may therefore be free to create the model in the comfort of his own home. To avoid the unpleasantness of approaching the lab workers, his wife can volunteer to bring the specimen cup into the lab on his behalf.

The fear of the results is the next obstacle. Many guys associate their sense of sexual prowess and the caliber of their sperm with being genuinely masculine. A guy can be stopped in his tracks even by the prospect of receiving a poor semen analysis result as a negative diagnostic.

How can a lady bring up the topic without starting a dispute or a disagreement? It is wise to approach this subject delicately. A woman ought to think about it from his point of view: the embarrassment, worry about the consequences, and the potential assault on his masculinity. These problems can be extremely genuine and make a man hesitate. According to studies, it can take a man several months after one has been ordered to get a semen analysis.

It is possible to talk about getting a semen analysis from a financial perspective. The test is frequently among the most affordable fertility tests available, and insurance might pay for it. The couple may feel more at ease knowing what to expect from the results.

But there is a real chance that the issue could be with the male. Sadly, women sometimes have to use caution in this circumstance and refrain from openly expressing their worry that they could have a semen problem. Here, a kind and non-accusatory tone are appropriate. It's vital to avoid placing blame at this time because the diagnosis is shared in 20–40% of cases.

2. She might not be ovulating, and he might have a low sperm count. Whatever the cause of the issue, they are in it together as a pair.

Using the services of a counselor, particularly a fertility counselor, may be beneficial to address the deeper marital concerns thoroughly. Of course, men unwilling to speak with a fertility counselor may have hidden worries about participating in fertility treatments. Men who are not very forthcoming about the process could perceive counseling as putting them in a comparable vulnerable position to having the testing done. The fertility counselor might take the initiative if a woman successfully persuades her partner to attend counseling so that it is not perceived as an attack coming from her.

Additionally, it's essential to approach the process with an open mind; the counselor isn't there to side with either party but rather to assist them in managing their emotions so they can make wise decisions. The counselor can highlight the variety of problems connected to infertility. About all diagnoses, men are involved roughly 50% of the time. Additionally, there is a strong likelihood that the issue affects both men and women. Individual and joint counseling sessions with a psychotherapist can both be helpful.

How can a woman encourage a man to view himself as a true collaborator in the conception process? The fact that "the pair" is now a woman and her doctor can surely make men feel excluded. An additional test of his masculinity and function in the relationship occurs when the doctor unexpectedly assumes the role of the one who will make her pregnant. Consider this and offer to incorporate him as much as possible. A brilliant place to start is by using a Conception Kit that you may use at home.

3. If he chooses, the man can participate in cycle planning using the Conception Kit. The fact that the couple engages in sexual activity rather than just gathering sperm in a restroom is the finest part. The semen is obtained using the kit, placed in a non-spermicidal, non-latex condom, and then transferred to a cervical silicone cap that the woman wears. You can also use The Conception Kit to ease the man's hesitation before getting a semen analysis. It might

encourage a hesitant couple to get going sooner!

The male might not want to participate in the procedure any further. Women are more likely to dive in and learn everything they can, following their cycles meticulously and keeping an eye out for any conception indicators. Men adopt a more simple, straightforward strategy. The man and the woman can complement one another by realizing that these differences can be a strength. It's crucial to refrain from demanding that he respond to the difficulties of trying to conceive in the same manner as she does. Don't push him too hard; let him be himself and accept him for who he is.

www.ingramcontent.com/pod-product-compliance
Lightning Source LLC
Chambersburg PA
CBHW050320220526
45465CB00005B/2061